THE HEROES HISTORY

The undying story
of the very last heroes/ heroin

BY

HARVEY VICTOR

TABLE OF CONTENT

DESCRIPTION

The psychology of heroism may not be nicely understood, however many experts do trust that it's far feasible for human beings to learn to be heroes. The following are only some of the important characteristics that researchers have ascribed to heroes.Situation for the nicely-being of others.In keeping with researchers, empathy, and compassion for others are key variables that make a contribution to heroic conduct.Individuals who rush in to help others within the face of danger and adversity accomplish that because they definitely care about the safety and properly being of other humans.In its earliest use, the word hero turned into carried out nearly solely to a man. The corresponding word heroine became and nonetheless is reserved for a girl. Hero is still sometimes used to refer mainly to a person. british heroes and heroines. But hero is now taken into consideration to be a gender impartial phrase, and is also increasingly more used to refer to a female: a list of yankee heroes; joan of arc, a french hero. Inside the experience "the most important person in a story, play, and many others.," a hero is male and a heroine is woman: margaret is the novel's heroine.Greek mathematician who wrote on mechanics and invented many water pushed and steam pushed machines. He additionally developed a way for figuring out the area of a triangle.

Researchers propose that heroes are not simply compassionate and being concerned; they've a knack for being capable of see things from the angle of others. they could "walk a mile in any other guy's shoes," so to talk.Once they come upon a scenario in which an individual is in want, they are without delay capable of see themselves in that identical state of affairs and see what desires to be carried out to assist.Heroes have beneficial competencies and strengths.Actually, having the education or physical potential to deal with a disaster can also play a prime function in whether or no longer humans come to be heroes.In conditions where could-be rescuers lack the expertise or sheer bodily electricity to make a distinction, human beings are less probable to assist or are more likely to locate less direct methods to take action. And in many cases, this approach is probably exceptional; after all, human beings senselessly dashing into a risky situation can pose even greater problems for rescue workers.People who are skilled and succesful, consisting of people with first resource training and revel in, are more prepared and capable of step up whilst their skills are wanted.

Heroes have a robust ethical compass:Consistent with

heroism researchers zimbardo and franco, heroes have two important qualities that set them apart from non-heroes: they stay by way of their values and they're inclined to undergo non-public threat to guard those values.

Chapter 1.The primary warfare: the monster grendel

In denmark, king hrothgar suggestions. Certainly one of his many achievements is the improvement of a splendid mead corridor, known as heorot. This large corridor is the king's throne-room, and a place for feasts. However the festivities don't very last lengthy. One night time, evil arrives at heorot within the form of a prowling monster, grendel. He lurks outside at the same time as the men eat and drink inside the corridor. And after they go to sleep, grendel movements. The monster grabs 30 men from their beds and drags their mangled corpses again to his lair. The subsequent night time time, grendel actions once more. And however.Night time time after night time time, for 12 years, the humans at heorot live in worry. They're helpless and hopeless, as their prayers to the pagan gods circulate unanswered. However then every other traveler arrives at the corridor – a young prince and warrior who's sailed throughout the sea. His name is beowulf.

He tells the king that he and his guys have heard of the relentless attacks at heorot. They've come to offer their assist. Defeating grendel acquired't be easy, says beowulf. And he's privy to that he risks finishing up as the monster's next meal. But the younger prince isn't afraid. He places his believe in god. "fate goes as fate should," says beowulf. At ultimate, for the primary time in years, there's a glimmer of desire at the king's corridor.That night time, after a heat welcome and a hearty night meal, beowulf and his men brace themselves for grendel's arrival. Inside the middle of the night, the door swings open. Grendel paces the room, gleefully eying up the sleeping warriors. What he doesn't apprehend is that beowulf is awake and searching.

Then, the monster moves. Grendel sinks his claws and tooth into one of the napping men. He bites right down to the bone, ingesting the man or woman's blood and devouring him piece thru piece, till there's not some thing left. Grendel then creeps towards beowulf's mattress, organized to seize his next sufferer. But rather, it's beowulf who seizes him, grabbing maintain of the monster's arm.And so the fight starts offevolved. No guns, just pure physical power as beowulf and grendel conflict, stumbling and crashing thru the hall. Benches are knocked over, and the very timbers of the wonderful corridor begin to shake.Grendel lets out a blood-curdling wail of pain. Now not due to the sword blows from beowulf's guys, who've rushed to their leader's protection. The swords don't leave a scratch. Great beowulf himself is capable of injure the monster, the usage of his bare palms.He maintains grendel locked in his effective grip till a wound seems on the monster's shoulder. It receives large and large till the sinews split and the bone breaks. Beowulf rips off grendel's whole arm.

The conflict is over. Mortally wounded, grendel staggers far from the hall, leaving a route of gore in his wake. He returns to his lair inside the marsh, wherein the water turns purple with blood. And there, the monster breathes his very last.Lower back at heorot, the humans are jubilant. Way to beowulf's excellent energy and heroism, they not need to stay in worry.The following morning, the hall is repaired, and a grisly new ornament is introduced – grendel's arm now hangs from the eaves of the roof. Overwhelmed with remedy and gratitude, the king tells beowulf that he now considers him a son. He showers him with items, which incorporates weapons, armor, horses, and a spectacular gold neck chain. Spirits are excessive that night time, due to the fact the guys dinner party and have an amazing time. Little do they recognize that outside, a today's threat is lurking.

Chapter 2.The second warfare: grendel's mother

It seems the monster had a mom.Grief-troubled, grendel's mother is now out for revenge. That night time she entails heorot. And at the identical time because the men are sound asleep, she pounces. She kills a man – the king's closest companion – then flees lower back to the marsh.The following morning, beowulf – who modified into dozing some place else that night time – is summoned lower back to heorot. The king is deeply distressed through the murder of his pal and the advent of another danger. However beowulf tells him to be strong. This is the time for movement, not mourning. He reassures the king that he'll find and kill grendel's mother. He'll avenge the individual's dying, and store heorot from chance once more.

So beowulf and his men experience off to the marsh searching out grendel's mom. He's been warned that the lake in which she lives is a haunted, desolate area, averted with the resource of flora and fauna. And at night time time, some thing strange and mysterious takes region there – the water burns.While beowulf arrives on the lake, it seems to be even more sinister than he have become expecting. The pinnacle of the individual killed with the useful resource of grendel's mom lies on the floor. And the water and surrounding cliffs are swarming with reptilian monsters. Status at the shore, beowulf fingers for the combat. All all all over again, he's organized to fulfill his future.

"with this sword," he says, "i am capable of advantage glory or die." and with that, he dives into the depths of the lake.Beowulf is going down … down … down. Hours skip earlier than he catches sight of the bottom. However in advance than he can get there, grendel's mother grabs him. , beowulf finds himself being dragged into her lair, at the same time as sea monsters attack him on all factors. In the gloomy underwater cavern, beowulf starts offevolved offevolved his 2nd most essential war.To his dismay, his sword turns out to be vain towards grendel's mother. He inns to stopping alongside along along with his naked hands, certainly as he did together with her son. They're rapid in the midst of a violent wrestling suit. Then grendel's mom takes out a knife. But beowulf is covered via his chaln mail – for now.

After which he spots some difficulty inside the cavern: a huge, heavy sword. It's so large, it seems to had been made for giants. No regular man can also want to wield it. But that is beowulf. He is taking the sword, and with a single blow, slices through his opponent's neck.The monster's mom is useless.However one decapitation isn't enough. Catching sight of grendel's corpse in each different a part of the cavern, beowulf cuts off his head too. In the meantime, up above, the guys are expecting beowulf's pass lower back, and turning into increasingly disturbing. After they see the blood in the water, masses of them lose desire and depart. But the few who continue to be are quickly rewarded with an unforgettable sight.

Beowulf emerges from the lake and swims to the shore. He's carrying trophies from the battle. One is the hilt of the large sword. It's all that's left, due to the fact the blade of the sword has melted, burned up via the hot blood of the monster. The opposite trophy is the pinnacle of the monster himself.Beowulf reasons pretty a scene on his pass decrease lower back to the corridor, dragging grendel's head throughout the ground. It's a image of triumph, says beowulf. Over again, there are feasts and celebrations at heorot. At closing, they'll be comfy.Even as it's time for beowulf to go away, the king offers the younger hero greater gadgets and lavishes him with reward. No longer best has beowulf saved them from hazard, but he's additionally united worldwide places – the geats and the danes. Because the guys encompass, the king breaks down in tears. He loves beowulf like a son. And deep down, he is aware about that they'll in no manner meet head to head another time.Now, beowulf's destiny is taking him some place else – again to his home in geatland in what's now southern sweden.

Chapter 3.The third conflict: the dragon

Agree with it or no longer, lower back home, beowulf turned into once taken into consideration a weakling. However the younger warrior has now validated himself. After returning to geatland, beowulf sooner or later becomes a king himself. He's a sturdy and smart chief, who regulations properly for fifty years. But then a brand new hazard emerges in beowulf's state – a ferocious, hearth-breathing dragon.The dragon has been provoked by a robbery. A person stole a golden cup from its treasure hoard. Enraged, the dragon emerges from its cave and scorches everything in sight. It does this night after night, wreaking havoc all through the kingdom, and even burning down beowulf's home.Beowulf realizes that he's approximately to face his final battle. But after all the dangers he's faced over time, he's no longer afraid. He's equipped for this. As he prepares to take at the dragon, he tells his men that this is his conflict to fight. He'll combat for the distinction of prevailing, even though it outcomes in his demise.

Beowulf approaches the dragon's cave. From the hole comes a blaze of flames. After which the dragon itself, in a burst of fire and rage. Again and again once more, beowulf slashes with his sword. However it doesn't cut via the dragon's scales. Along with his weapon failing him, it appears that evidently beowulf might also have in the end met his healthy. His men, who've been watching from a distance, all flee in terror. All except one. A younger warrior, wiglaf, is the handiest one to help beowulf. Moved by pity, and gratitude for the whole thing the king has finished for him, wiglaf joins the struggle. The 2 guys combat side by way of side. While the dragon's breath burns up wiglaf's protect, he shares beowulf's. For a while, they manage to guard themselves, however their swords do little damage.Then the dragon lunges, and bites into beowulf's neck. Seeing the blood pouring down beowulf's frame, wiglaf realizes the situation is now critical. He strikes the dragon again, and this time the sword goes proper into the beast's stomach. In spite of his injury, beowulf then summons up his ultimate last strength. He's taking a knife from his belt and plunges it deep into the dragon's facet.Beowulf has added the very last blow – the fatal wound. The dragon dies. Now, the warfare is over, however so is beowulf's life.Reeling from ache and nausea, he senses the dragon's poison festering inside him. And he is aware of that death is close to. Wiglaf enables beowulf to do away with his helmet and has a tendency to his wounds. In his loss of life moments, beowulf reflects on his lifestyles. He may not have a son and heir but he's taking consolation from understanding that for 50 years, he changed into a great, sturdy chief.Beowulf removes the gold collar from his neck and gives it to wiglaf. And then, taking into account his family and ancestry, beowulf utters his ultimate phrases. "they're all gone," he says. "my complete clan has gone to their doom. Now, it's my flip to observe."

The people of geatland mourn beowulf's demise foreseeing dark instances beforehand. Without their king to shield them, assaults from their enemies at the moment are inevitable.In keeping with beowulf's wishes, his body is burned on a good sized pyre. Because the smoke rises as much as the heavens, a lady weeps, imagining the destiny of the state – a grim imaginative and prescient of rampaging enemies, piles of our bodies, and slavery. After the funeral, the geats construct a burial mound on a headland. Beowulf's tomb is so imposing that it's seen from a ways away at sea. In a very last ceremony, 12 warriors journey around the tomb, mourning their leader. He was so type and sturdy, with such ambition!

Of all the kings on earth, beowulf changed into the best.Beowulf is a story poem set in scandinavia in the 6th century. It tells the tale of a heroic warrior, prince beowulf.As a younger guy, beowulf travels to denmark and gives his help on the mead corridor of king hrothgar. For years, the hall has been terrorized with the aid of an evil monster, grendel. A dramatic conflict takes region, and beowulf manages to mortally wound grendel with his naked palms. The subsequent night time, grendel's devastated mother assaults the corridor in revenge and kills a close pal of the king. Beowulf hunts down grendel's mother in her underwater lair. Every other violent conflict ensues, and he kills her with a large sword. The king's hall is now secure at closing. Beowulf sails again to his domestic in geatland, wherein he will become king.

Fifty years later, beowulf is positioned to the take a look at once more, when his country is attacked by means of a ferocious dragon. In a very last epic conflict, beowulf kills the dragon. But shortly later on, he dies from his accidents. Beowulf's frame is burned on a pyre and an outstanding burial mound is constructed in his memory. The story ends with the people of geatland mourning their chief – the best the world has ever recognised.

Chapter 4.Discover the psychological power of classic heroic mythology.

When Joseph Campbell traveled through Europe as a college student in his mid-1920s, he got to hear first-hand the philosophies and myths of other cultures. This led to a lifelong fascination with comparative mythology.Having studied cultures from all over the world, including Asian, African, European, Polynesian, and Native American, Campbell found that their stories had more than just common thematic elements. Also, the characters in these stories tended to go through three different stages. They left their communities, endured a series of hardships, became enlightened beings, and then returned home to share their newfound wisdom and new powers.

These stages became known as Monomyths, or the quintessential hero's journey, and the structure described by Campbell has inspired countless storytellers since. Perhaps most notorious is the fact that George Lucas could only finish the first script for a Star Wars movie after reading Campbell's work.In this Blink of his, we take you through every stage and milestone in the protagonist's journey, revealing why this story has remained true for centuries.When we embark on the hero's journey, it is important to know that we are dealing with mythology, a world full of symbols and metaphors. Campbell notes that this is basically the same world as our unconscious dream state. After all, these myths are products of the fertile human imagination and were often created in response to the deepest fears and concerns of our ancestors. Indeed, after studying the records of famous psychoanalysts Sigmund Freud and Carl Jung, Campbell found that the dreams of modern people were still full of the same symbols and conflicts that make up the monomyth.So why is this important? Because the hero's journey is as much about revealing inner truths as it is about slaying dragons. Along the way, the hero inevitably discovers that he had everything he needed to overcome adversity and find enlightenment at all times.So let's start at the beginning - with the first leg of the hero's journey - known as the start. The start consists of five stages or subsections in which the hero leaves the comfort of his ordinary environment and crosses the threshold into a more dreamlike world.

The first stage is known as the "Call to Adventure". This is the moment when the hero is confronted with something that distracts him from his usual routine. It can be a mysterious stranger standing by the side of the road or something as fantastic as a talking animal. In some cases, the hero can glimpse a hidden world. In any case, symbolically speaking, this encounter is also a momentary personal revelation. The hero realizes that the call to adventure speaks of something special that has been repressed within him - which is why the hero often encounters this development with a mixture of fear, uncertainty and restlessness.From the beginning, we have a conflict which brings us to the second stage: the "rejection of the appeal". Often we don't want to leave the comfort of our normal life. We don't want to venture into a new and potentially dangerous world. Or, more accurately, we don't want to face that fearful and repressed element within us.

But for the heroes who finally answer the call, there's encouragement in the third phase, known as "Supernatural Aid." This often comes in the form of a mercurial elder or mentor who gives the hero the advice and protective amulets he needs to begin his journey. This is the character who first mentions that the hero has a "destiny" that he must fulfill—that the repressed element within him is a gift that must be unlocked. The mentor figure could very well be the fairy godmother of children's lore. But more often than not, they're a mix of friendly and menacing. Yes, they serve as a guard and guide, but also as someone who lures the hero into danger. In Dante's Inferno, this is the character of Virgil. In Goethe's Faust, it is Mephistopheles who sends the hero out to face the trials and tribulations that await him.In essence, this supernatural guide leads the hero across the frontier into a realm of darkness and mystery, which is why the fourth step is referred to as "crossing the first threshold". At this point, the hero tends to encounter another menacing figure: a "guard of the threshold" who challenges and repels intruders. Countless mythologies are populated by terrifying characters and monsters that are found on the edge of unknown forests, oceans, jungles or deserts.Thus we arrive at the fifth and last step of the starting phase: the "belly of the whale". Here the hero is consumed by the unknown. The first impression at this point is that instead of capturing the power of the mysterious dark world, the hero is defeated and killed by it.

Death is one of the most important parts of the journey. In all the mythologies of the world there is a common idea that in order to reach a higher state of being, the old form must cease to exist. Before the hero can continue their journey of transformation, their previous unenlightened form must be extinguished.

Chapter 5.The inauguration

After leaving the house, crossing the threshold and emerging from the belly of the whale like a metaphorical newborn, the hero can now embark on the second stage of the journey: initiation.

This is the part of the hero mythos where the transformation into a powerful new being really begins. It begins with the sixth stage of the journey, the "path of trials".In countless stories, the hero is subjected to a series of trials that will test both his resolve and his abilities. Consider Psyche trying to win Cupid's love. Cupid's mother, Venus, had him sort through a vast pile of grain and seeds, gather golden wool from a poisonous wild sheep, then fetch a bottle of water from the top of a mountain inhabited by a dragon. . Each challenge was tougher and more deadly than the last. But without fail, Psyche got help at just the right time—that's another common trope. An army of ants helped her sort through the grain pile. A magic rod helped her collect wool. An eagle helped her get water. During their trials, the hero tends to humble themselves by the gift of help. This further eliminates the ego and focuses their energies on the path to enlightenment. Often the help they receive points them in some way towards their new higher purpose.

After overcoming the obstacles on the path of trials, the next step - the seventh of the whole journey - is the "Meeting with the Goddess". Here, the hero faces the queen of the world. If you thought of the hero's journey as a circle, that would be the lowest point - but it's also the high point of the quest. From there, things can get a bit complex and contradictory. This makes sense: in many cultures, as well as in some Eastern philosophies, the ability to reconcile the conflicting facts of life is one of the keys to enlightenment.In "Encounter with the Goddess", the hero is confronted with a figure that represents all women and the creative power that accompanies them. She is the sister, the lover, the wife. She is both a kind and loving mother and a controlling and disciplined mother. This part of the journey is about the hero understanding both the womb and the grave - two things that go hand in hand.Then comes the eighth stage, called "the seductive woman". How willing is the hero to give up the earthly pleasures he has known to attain the higher powers of a more enlightened being? This is another test the hero must pass.In the ninth stage, the hero is then confronted with the other parent: "Reconciliation with the father". Similar to the encounter with the Goddess, this stage involves letting go of any remaining dependencies or conceptions, such as the superego and the id, that might stand in the way of achieving transcendence. This is also the stage in which the hero must reconcile the potentially conflicting ideas of God and sin. It is about finding harmony in contradiction, letting go and moving forward.The tenth and penultimate step of the initiatory stage is called "apotheosis," which means deification, or the act of becoming a god. Having faced the Goddess and the Father, the hero has achieved an understanding of the world - and the transcendence and enlightenment that go with it. In Buddhist terms, the hero becomes a bodhisattva, or "one whose essence is enlightenment". Things like fear, pain, and pleasure, as well as concepts like "good" and "bad," become obsolete concerns. In Hinduism he is called jivan mukta, "one who is liberated in life". The hero is now desireless, compassionate, and wise. The ego is completely dissolved to the point that even enemies are loved.

The initiation phase ends with the eleventh stage, the "ultimate blessing". It was the achievement of the goal that started the journey. Everything that happened before prepared the hero for this moment. Given the transcendent state they are in now, the blessing is ultimately captured with grace and ease.So what comes next? Aren't we done? Not enough. In the final section, we look at the third and final leg of the hero's journey.The hero's journey is not about selfish desires. The emphasis is on sharing grace, wisdom, and the enlightenment gained. After all, a hero is someone who helps others. So to do that we have to go back to the communities we left. That's right, regression is the name of the last leg of the journey. But the first part of this stage, which is the entire twelfth step, is called "refusal to return."

Sometimes the hero is simply overwhelmed by the ecstasy of transcendence and cannot return home. Other characters may wonder what it means to return – is it even possible for those who understand the depth of the gift? Still others may try to take it a step further and extend the withdrawal phase. But to actually continue their journey, they have to turn around and go home. This return usually begins with the thirteenth step, called "Magic Flight." You're probably familiar with stories where the ultimate reward is protected by sleeping giants or other menacing guardians. So when a hero grabs a blessing, a chase begins, often involving heroic feats. There may be more magical obstacles, but the hero overcomes them - perhaps with the help of some supernatural power. In other stories, the main character needs help to get home, so the fourteenth step is called "delivery from outside". Perhaps the hero enters a state of blissful euphoria. Or they may be trapped or imprisoned somewhere. Take the example of the Japanese goddess Amaterasu, who before leaving on a journey leaves a message that reads, "If I don't return by a certain time, come and get me." That's exactly what happened, and saving Amaterasu became his own heroic journey.Whether it is rescue or magical flight, the fifteenth step is to "cross the threshold." Here we explore what happens when everyone discovers that the characters are forever changed by their adventure. In the story of Rip Van Winkle, who returns home after 20 years of sleep, the main character is unrecognizable. People in his hometown consider him a suspicious and potentially dangerous stranger. Therefore, reintegration into society and sharing the ecstasy of enlightenment with an unaware and unprepared society can be one of the biggest challenges of the entire journey.

The sixteenth step is called "Lord of the Two Realms." The hero finds a way to cross the abyss and demonstrates this mastery. This moment is so compelling that it appears in the founding stories of many religions. This is when the unenlightened see the manifestation of the hero's power and immediately realize its meaning. It is often terrifying to witness, but the depth of this divine power is undeniable.Finally, we come to the seventeenth and final part of our journey: "The Freedom to Live." Sounds good, right? This stage embodies the steadfast nature of the enlightened hero that we talked about in the "Fengshen" stage: not to be afraid of death. No attachment to pain or pleasure. The ability to see all things as equally valuable parts of the whole.But now that the heroes have shared this gift, they too can live truly carefree and free – knowing that what's inside them affects everyone else's insides.

Chapter 6.Select energy over pressure to transform your global

In today's speedy paced international, it's smooth to sense crushed. Out of doors forces like politics, society, and the economy shape our lives, regularly making us experience powerless.

But what if you did have energy, and this strength within you helped you create effective modifications within the global? Contrary to what human beings believe, energy does not rely upon external manipulation; as a substitute, it is rooted in our capability to influence and rework our reviews. And it's handy to every person.Electricity is not the same as force. Force would possibly appear to be a brief fix, however it is just a temporary solution, main to undesirable consequences. Strength, on the other hand, is a gradual burning fireplace that produces lasting results. You can use it to triumph over demanding situations and acquire dreams peacefully with none struggling or bloodshed. And you could additionally use it to locate 'sure' or 'no' solutions to even the maximum hard questions.So are you prepared to electricity up in your quality life? This blink will help you apprehend and harness your electricity efficiently so you can normalize transformation, innovation and collaboration via clean picks irrespective of who you are or what you do.

Stay Aware

To tap into your inner strength, you must first understand the role of your consciousness.Imagine your mind as a landscape with mountains and valleys. They represent different levels of consciousness. Some yearn for heights where love, peace and joy reign. So we are always looking for clarity and deeper understanding. Some stray into the lower realms where anger, shame, guilt, and other limiting thoughts prevent connection and remain in survival mode.

Now imagine this landscape as a scale from 1 to 1000. Each number represents a level of consciousness. According to the author, the shame that often leads us to self-destruction comes 20 years later. At 30, guilt sets in and it's easy to feel unworthy of being loved. When Fear reaches 100, we feel anxious and irritable all the time. But when you turn 200, you have the courage to face your fears and encourage yourself to take responsibility for your actions. As we climb the ladder, we find love that shines in the 500 and opens us to compassion and connection. At this level, our lives can change for the better. And when we reach the age of 700, we can finally cross the threshold of enlightenment and touch the pinnacle of human and spiritual consciousness.

Individuals, communities and even nations can have a positive impact on the world if they act in a high state of mind. For what? Well, the higher we are on the ladder of consciousness, the more we embrace our inner forces and the further away we are from destructive forces. Therefore, we look at the world more broadly, meet life's challenges with grace and creativity, and act as a positive ripple effect in reality.It is therefore clear that raising the level of awareness is a top priority. But awareness is only the beginning. If force is the movement of a car, consciousness is the car we drive. And we know that every car needs fuel. The time has come to unravel the phenomenon of intention, the fuel of power.

set wise intentions

Imagine starting your day with a clear goal. You know what you want to achieve and are goal driven. This clarity is the essence of intention, which guides our actions and shapes our reality.

When we set our intentions, we direct our lives, focus our energy on what matters most, and direct our destiny in the direction we want. Powerful intentions create waves of positive influence not only in our reality, but also in the reality of those around us.Clarity is what makes intent really strong. Being aware of your state of consciousness makes it easier to understand what you want. This clarity allows us to set wise intentions. Think of them as guiding stars that help you navigate life's ups and downs and achieve goals you never thought were yours.Suppose you want to improve your health. To do that, you need a clear intention to exercise regularly and eat well. This intention guides your daily choices and encourages you to stay true to purpose. You may not notice it now, but over time you will notice a dramatic improvement in your health. By doing so, you encourage your friends and family to make healthy lifestyle choices.Or imagine you are an entrepreneur dreaming of a business that benefits your community. Perhaps you're looking to start a business that offers fair wages and supports local initiatives. This intent guides every critical business decision, from the people we hire to the equipment we use. As your business grows, your community may see and recognize your intentions and be encouraged to join your cause.Of course, the boundless power of intention doesn't just inspire personal dreams. It also inspires group activities that ultimately shape our common world.Of course, life always gives us lemons. What happens when, despite your best intentions, you encounter unexpected difficulties? This is where surrender comes into play. It's the basis of true power, and we'll learn how to do that later.

master the art of renunciation

Surrender may look like surrender or surrender, but it's actually strength training. It's about letting go, trusting the flow of life, and opening up new possibilities. In today's fast-paced world, we often find ourselves clinging to control, wanting to know what happens next, and planning everything out. But life is unpredictable and sometimes the best way to deal with uncertainty is to let go and trust the process. Surrender is therefore a gateway to personal growth, allowing us to experience profound change in the face of adversity.But rest assured, giving up is not the same as giving up. Many of us have a hard time letting go of it because many people don't know the difference. In fact, giving up does not mean giving up on our dreams and goals. Instead, we recognize that something more is at work and let that guide us. We step into the unknown with courage and curiosity, believing that we will find the way. There is no better evidence of the power of incarceration than the story of Nelson Mandela, who spent 27 years in prison fighting for the freedom of his people. During his imprisonment, Mandela mastered the art of surrender, let go of resentment and hatred, and focused instead on forgiveness and unity. This shift in perspective allowed him to endure a prison sentence and emerge as a leader who helped end apartheid in South Africa.

How about going somewhere with a more relaxed atmosphere? Now, imagine that you are an artist whose creativity feels stunted. I've tried everything to break through, but nothing seems to work. Only by surrendering to circumstances can you let go of expectations and just create without judgment. Suddenly inspiration strikes and you are immersed in the real work. Surrender, after all, is about embracing the unknown and trusting yourself in your journey. When we let go of control of our circumstances, we open ourselves up to new possibilities, opportunities, and growth. In this moment of acceptance, we discover our inner strength and resilience and are able to face challenges with grace and courage.

Chapter 7 Parent the truth in any scenario with carried out kinesiology

With excellent strength comes high-quality obligation. So whether or not you're a college instructor or an internationally diagnosed politician, you can alternate your environment and the sector for the higher. But you may't wield power without fact in a international rife with false data, opinions and beliefs.So how do you tell what is authentic from fake? What if there were a technique that might provide you with the solution, all the time.In line with the author there may be, and it's referred to as implemented kinesiology.Applied kinesiology is a realistic answer allowing you to determine your truth amidst data overload and conflicting opinions with your muscle mass. That's right: you may examine the right statement, perception or even meals sorts for you with just your frame!How is that this viable. Properly, we have dr. George goodheart to thank. This exquisite modern physiotherapist dove into muscle-testing strategies in 1971 and made a wild discovery: muscle energy or weakness is connected to the fitness of specific frame organs, acupuncture meridians and bodily reactions to one of a kind stimuli. Photograph this: the deltoid muscles of humans with hypoglycemia or low blood glucose all at once weakened once they tasted sugar. Crazy, proper? This breakthrough brought about carried out kinesiology, an remarkable device for determining how one of a kind substances have an effect on our our bodies.

Now, permit's speak about dr. John diamond, the psychiatrist who took kinesiology to a new level by way of growing behavioral kinesiology. He explored how sensory and mental factors like art, song and emotional pressure impacted sufferers. Later studies could discover that the frame responded accurately even when the conscious thoughts had no clue what become being examined. Thanks to those splendid insights, the author believes you can use kinesiology to discern how true any declaration is to you primarily based in your inner experience of harmony.Give this a attempt: clutch a friend, amplify one arm, and withstand their downward stress in your wrist. Think about a assertion whilst they take a look at your arm's electricity. If it is a 'no,' your arm goes susceptible; if it's a 'sure,' it remains sturdy. Observe the difference when thinking about someone you love versus a person you fear. It really is carried out kinesiology for you.Mastering to inform reality from falsehood takes time and exercise, however its rewards are really worth our regular efforts. As we sharpen our minds to suss matters out higher and faster, we can seamlessly navigate lifestyles's complexities, leverage truth to make significant choices and lead with strength.

He ruled by force, not power

Everyone knows when they see strong leadership. The signs are clear. It is always about control, coercion and manipulation. Threat managers often focus only on the short term. Think of all the villains you see in movies and in real life. Often their only motive is to relieve hidden anger, guilt, or shame. Not surprisingly, their actions often backfire and the consequences of their actions can undermine team morale, trust and cohesion. On the other hand, strong leaders are based on influence, inspiration and authority. Power-hungry leaders create an environment where people feel valued, motivated and engaged. This enables collaboration and innovation to thrive, ensuring positive long-term outcomes for all involved. Historical examples of this contrast can be seen in the leadership styles of Mahatma Gandhi and Adolf Hitler. Gandhi's strong leadership inspired millions to achieve India's independence through non-violent civil disobedience. His vision brings people together and promotes lasting change. Instead, Hitler used violence, coercion and fear to control his followers, with dire consequences and great human suffering. The same management principles apply to business. It is enough to remember the story of Sam Walton, the founder of Walmart. While building a retail empire, Walton has focused on service and human values, creating a positive and supportive work environment that embraces customer interactions. This Walmart employee showed his leadership skills. Unlike other big box stores with cold, insensitive and ill-informed employees, Walmart employees are friendly, helpful and most importantly, they are there. Walton realized early on that a person's energy field in the workplace can lead to avoidance of hostile and confrontational environments, as well as friendship and loyalty with customers. It's no surprise that Walmart is a powerful company. A brand with a soul. By choosing nonviolence over violence, leaders can create an environment where people can thrive, innovate, and thrive. So what kind of leader do you want to be? A strong leader who controls and limits? Or are you a strong leader who inspires and motivates you? Remember that everyone around you will feel the impact of your choices.overcome conflict peacefully.

Conflict is an inevitable part of life. Disagreements and misunderstandings always arise between people everywhere, whether in personal relationships or in world politics. Because, firstly, people are different and always have different mindsets. What if conflict didn't always have to be exhausting? What if we could change our approach to conflict resolution instead of using force? True strength lies in the quest for compassion, understanding, and harmony. Approaching conflict resolution from this perspective creates space for healing, growth, and lasting resolution. Imagine two neighbors getting into a heated argument over a common fence. Neighbors choose to use force and threaten legal action to escalate the situation. Another Neighbor embraces the gentle nature of true power and invites partners to discuss their problems openly, seeking mutually beneficial solutions. This powerful approach resolves conflicts and strengthens bonds between neighbors. The same principle applies to other social areas of our lives. We can transform our relationships, our workplaces, and our communities by choosing power over power. When we approach conflict with a sincere desire for empathy and understanding, we foster true growth.Imagine a world where conflict resolution relies on real power. People unite to overcome their differences and seek solutions that benefit all parties involved. Such a world is based on harmony, cooperation and progress. So we can continue to use force to resolve conflicts, or we can harness the transformative potential of real power. By choosing power and the higher states of mind needed to activate it, we open the door to a world of greater understanding, compassion, and unity, And it's a world worth chasing.Power drives personal growth, sets an example, and enables conflict resolution. But doing so is like being at a crossroads. Mastering it always requires a great deal of introspection and insight into your surroundings.By harnessing power and the ideas that govern it, we can create paradigm shifts that change the world. It may sound mundane, but it is true that each of us has the ability to find harmony and compassion in our environment.Now, the right question is, what if we choose power over strength in every aspect of our lives? Now is the best time to find out. Because it can be done.

Chapter 8.Recognize spiritual fundamentalism through a true crime tale

In 1984, brenda lafferty and her daughter, erica, had been brutally murdered by ron and dan lafferty. The brothers had been a part of a fundamentalist mormon institution – once they decided to kill their sister-in-law and niece, they have been acting on a revelation they believed to be from god. In this blink to jon krakauer's below the banner of heaven, you'll discover no longer simply a crime story, however also an evaluation of spiritual extremism. A content material warning earlier than we begin: this blink includes radical perspectives and image violence, so please proceed with warning.

divine revelation

It was no ordinary meeting. It was a gathering of saints, the most zealous saints. On that day, April 5, 1984, they met to confirm the revelations they had received from God. But even these fearless crusaders were shocked by what God had revealed to Ron Rafferty. The nine members of the Onia

Prophet School split. Watson and Dan Rafferty sided with their brother Ron, who had a divine revelation. The rest went fine.As we now know, the kidnapping revelation was beyond doubt. God commanded Ron Rafferty to kill his brother's wife, children, and two close friends. These people have interfered with God's work.Surprisingly, Ron's friends were astonished. Bernard Brady was so surprised that he expressed his concerns in an affidavit just in case.Dan Rafferty thought about it, questioned it, and acknowledged its revelation. As the weeks passed, his support turned into a sincere conviction. Dan soon began receiving revelations of his own. He began to understand his role in Ron's plan.

Ron was the mouth of God, Dan was the hand of God. It was Dan who was chosen to wield the supreme sword. His family, they told his brother Allen that his wife and children had to leave home. Allen was furious. He told his brothers that he would protect Brenda and young Erica even at the cost of his life. Brenda, a bright and outspoken 24-year-old woman who gave up a promising career in journalism to marry Allen. Allen never told her wife about this discovery. During the discussion, Ron and Dan openly discussed the sinister details of the plan in their mother's dining room. Her submissive wife Claudine, who had been repeatedly abused by Ron and Dan's father, did not move her eyelids. Her husband died of diabetes because he hated conventional medicine.After a backlash from close friends, Ron and Dan quit Prophet School. Their old friends are now demon children.The revelation Joseph Smith revealed in 1832 about the mighty One who will prepare the house of God before His Second Coming is coming soon. God chose Ron and Dan.In 1823, the angel Moroni led 17-year-old Joseph Smith to the Hills of Palmyra, New York. According to the angel, buried under the rock for 14,000 years were golden tablets containing the Bible written in Egyptian hieroglyphs. The plate would belong to Smith when he grew up and married.

Smith was in love with a girl named Emma Hale, but Emma's father was dissatisfied with their marriage. He didn't want Smith, a convicted swindler and fortune teller, to marry his beautiful daughter. The couple then fled. At Moroni's request, Smith visited Palmyra Hill every September

22nd. On his visit in 1827 Smith took his fiancée with him. They dressed in black and rode in a black wagon drawn by black horses.Having fulfilled the conditions set by the angel, Smith was given access to the Bible. Using spectacles given to him by Moroni, he read ancient documents aloud to his neighbor Martin Harris, who had taken over as scribe. When Moroni finished translating, he took up the gold plate and cup. And then the worst happened. Martin Harris borrowed the translated text and showed it to his shady wife...and he disappeared. It took Moroni some effort to return the plate. And this time Moroni offered no spectacle.So Smith relied on his own experience. He used an old technique he had learned during his treasure hunt. He placed a gold plate next to him and placed a saw-stone in his upturned hat, buried his head in it to block the light, and peered through the hole in the stone. He then read the English Bible to Emma and the other clerks.The team completed his translation in June 1829, but Smith could not afford the $3,000 advance for 5,000 copies of the Book of Mormon. In another vision, God revealed to Smith that Harris had to pay the printer. Harris has previously dealt with his wife's anger over their relationship with Smith. But even his wife could not stop him from doing God's work.Harris sold his farm to finance his publication, and Joseph Smith officially took up religion a week after the book's publication.

The Church of Jesus Christ of Latter-day Saints was born.A **weird**

humans

600 years earlier than the beginning of christ, a hebrew tribe left jerusalem and set sail for america.They were led by means of lehi, who subsequently picked his more youthful son, nephi, to lead the tribe. Lehi's choice didn't pass down properly with laman, the older son. Along along with his fans, laman's skin were given darker as he became extra evil.In keeping with smith's revelations, the evil faction have been ancestors of the local individuals. The lamanites killed all the nephites all however one, this is. This last nephite's call changed into mormon.Mormon's son, moroni, became the angel that exceeded joseph smith the golden plates at the holy web page mormons now call hill cumorah.

Smith's tale attracted derision from nearby newspapers and commentators – but it also attracted over one thousand converts in a single year from the region around palmyra. Smith declared his church the one and best real church.He additionally communicated with god on a regular basis – a ability his fans picked up. Smith's revelations, however, have been taken into consideration more sacred. They provided guidance for the status quo of his church and were posted in an reliable dogma which he titled the doctrine and covenants.Going through persecution in palmyra, smith acquired a revelation to steer god's selected to zion. The saints stopped briefly in kirtland, ohio, before settling in jackson county, missouri.

But tensions started to brew.To the people of jackson county, mormons had been an entitled institution: they preferred to exchange amongst themselves, voted as one bloc, and purchased up quite a few land around the location. The locals also disliked that those northerners preferred the abolition of slavery.Bloody clashes ensued, main to the deaths of many ladies and men on both facets. After one such conflict, smith supplied to sacrifice himself to set up peace.He changed into ordered to be shot alongside a number of his fans. However by way of this time, mormons had began to attract some public sympathy from individuals who idea they have been being persecuted for their religion. This deterred neighborhood government officers from taking place with the execution.Encouraged by means of a bribe, jail officials were given under the influence of alcohol and dozed off whilst the prisoners escaped. The saints crossed over into illinois and created a new agreement in the town of nauvoo, hancock county. It wasn't lengthy earlier than they enraged the locals again. However this time, the president, prophet, seer, and revelator of the church was starting to face some resistance from his home turf too.The street to fundamentalism

Officially, the mormon church rejects polygamy. However that's just one facet of joseph smith's legacy. Polygamy is practiced through limitless mormon sects. This department began underneath smith's personal roof.In nauvoo, smith began slumbering with different women. He secretly married a number of them, in what he known as "celestial marriages." guys had to marry as many ladies as they could to create offspring and populate god's earth, smith advised near friends.However strongly he felt about it, though, smith couldn't locate the courage to inform his spouse. He dropped some recommendations to look the response. It changed into poor. Understanding that the instances hadn't yet caught up with his audacious vision, he secretly canonized polygamy in section 132 of the doctrines and covenants as one of the crucial standards of mormonism.The street to salvation lay in those religious marriages. All and sundry who not noted this principle, character, would be damned.

In 1844, a church elder named william law sided with emma and threatened to expose smith in a newspaper article. Smith, appearing as mayor of nauvoo, raided regulation's office.Smith changed into arrested and locked up in carthage, illinois, but his enemies in hancock county broke into his cell and attacked him. He jumped out of the jail window and crashed to the ground, 20 ft beneath.Polygamy's time got here in 1852 while smith's successor, brigham younger, introduced smith's mystery precept to an meeting in salt lake town. Saints sympathizers were greatly surprised. However earlier than lengthy, it became the dogma and usual practice of the mainstream mormon church – the church wherein the lafferty brothers have been raised.

While ron lafferty and his brothers came throughout this revelation, they felt betrayed with the aid of the authorities in salt lake city. The church had compromised its ideas to make peace with the authorities of america. Not only had it renounced polygamy it had also allowed black humans to join the mormon church and priesthood. The lafferty better halves weren't glad with their husbands' revelation. They didn't like the reality that they had been discussing polygamy with antique men in distant communes, secretly marrying their stepdaughters, and sexually abusing their youngsters.As soon as the lafferty brothers followed mormon fundamentalism, they began counting on divine provision. Ron left his process and drove round without a license, often exceeding velocity limits to defy law enforcement officials. In his eyes, the regulation of god superseded the regulation of guy. He traveled to colorado metropolis in utah and bountiful in canada, and started experimenting with capsules and alcohol. His first wife had left with their children, so he commenced to take other wives.All people who opposed the chosen, smith had declared, was a toddler of the satan. Now not able to make their husbands see purpose, the lafferty wives turned to brenda, the youngest wife. Her interventions angered the lafferty guys.

On july 24, 1984, ron and dan lafferty parked their impala station wagon outdoor their brother allen's home in american fork. July 24 is pioneer day, which mormons have fun every year to commemorate the day their ancestors marched into utah territory returned in 1847.

Ron were given out and knocked on the front door no respond. He jumped returned into the car to enroll in dan and companions they'd been traveling around with.But as they drove far from allen's residence, dan all at once felt an urge. It changed into he, dan, that had been selected to perform this challenge. He turned the car around and drove lower back to allen's house.This time, brenda opened the door. He pressured his manner in and closed the door from inner. Then he attacked his sister-in-regulation. Ron entered the residence moments later and helped his brother subdue brenda, who passed out.Then dan walked into his niece erica's room. She changed into status in her crib, burbling and smiling at her uncle. Her uncle explained to the toddler that he became doing god's work, closed his eyes, after which slashed the child's throat with the tool god had chosen: a boning knife.Unfazed via what he'd simply finished, dan washed the blood off the knife. He walked lower back to the kitchen, where brenda lay immobile. He grabbed her by way of the hair, closed his eyes, and cut her throat too.

Sopping wet in blood, the brothers and their team drove to the home of their subsequent supposed victim: chloe low. She wasn't there she and her circle of relatives had determined to rejoice pioneer day away from american fork so that they stole some jewelry and cash, and destroyed chloe's collection of figurines. Chloe had angered the brothers via assisting their other halves. Richard stowe, their very last goal, had carried out the equal. However on their way to execute richard, they neglected a turn. And their partners decided they'd visible sufficient. They informed the brothers it wasn't god's will. That's why they'd missed the flip, their pals pleaded.Whilst their companions disappeared with their automobile, the brothers separated and reunited in reno, nevada. There, they depended on unfastened on line casino food and the generosity of strangers. A driving force let them sleep in his bus. Different times, unfastened casino chips could win them a meal.Sooner or later, they determined to test out a pal in circus circus casino. Once they didn't find her, they covered as much as eat on the on line casino's buffet. The police were ready. But ron and dan didn't resist – the whole lot they'd executed was the lord's work.

Whilst dan turned into mastering about the early mormon church, he determined blood atonement have been encouraged via joseph smith and his successor, brigham young. Spilling blood turned into satisfactory, they argued, if an unbeliever dedicated an unforgivable sin in opposition to a saint. Mormon legends like porter rockwell, additionally referred to as the destroying angel, killed many human beings on behalf of the church. Locked up in jail, ron had any other revelation: god had requested him to kill dan. He attempted to sneak up on his brother at the same time as he slept, however retreated whilst his brother awakened. On some other event, ron brutally attacked dan, who placed up no resistance.The brothers were separated and put in adjoining cells after this incident. Dan allow ron strangle him with a towel through his mobile. He suffered injuries but survived. Then it dawned on him: ron become the child of the devil. Dan now concept of himself because the prophet elijah, sent to earth to put together the way for christ.The brothers were convicted in separate trials dan to life in prison, ron to demise.

Chapter 9.Learn how to manage and even grow as a highly sensitive person.

Avoid parties? Do you feel compelled to sit at the event because leaving will hurt people's feelings.Do you get nervous when people see you doing what you usually do well? Do you stun people by coming up with great ideas?

Perhaps you are a very sensitive person. Contrary to popular belief, you are not shy. No spoilers for you either. You have an uncanny ability to pick up on nuances that others miss. Instead of worrying about this trait, you can help yourself and those around you by learning how to control and use this superpower. This short blink will tell you how.

Symptoms you're particularly touchy man or woman

Meet rob and rebecca. They're twins – fraternal, no longer identical.At age three, they grow to be big brother and huge sister, so a pleasant couple comes to care for the twins for some days before the new toddler comes domestic.Whilst rob walks into his parents' room and finds strangers, he's so terrified, he screams. Rebecca walks in, says hi, and rancid she goes, smiling.Rob's neither shy nor nerve-racking. He just sees, smells, and hears matters rebecca isn't prepared to soak up.He's inherited a enormously touchy frightened device. As he grows, he'll neglect maximum of what's befell in his early life – however his frame and subconscious will constantly do not forget.He'll spend more time processing occasions. His desires could be bright and could have loads to do with what's going on inside the real international. His dreams may even are expecting destiny activities with outstanding accuracy.

If that sounds such as you, you're most of the 20 percent of human beings with rob's superpower.What rob skilled whilst he noticed strangers in his dad and mom' bed wasn't always fear. It became records overload. He turned into just overstimulated.Exceptionally sensitive people, or hsps, will bitch about the quantity of tune at a bar. They'll capture the trace of a frown that asserts a colleague's wife hates christmas parties. They can judge the character of a florist with the aid of looking at how she arranges plants. These subtle clues can include splendid advantages. If you're an hsp, they will let you revel in the healthful sensory reports of laughter, tune, work, and sex.What you need to look out for is balance. Everybody has an most fulfilling arousal degree. Get above this threshold and you could revel in soreness, and, in extreme instances, paralysis or panic.

Of direction, everyone has a sensory threshold. The distinction here is that the extraordinarily touchy have decrease thresholds and won't be able to stand honking vehicles or huge crowds. A few might not even be capable of take small businesses for extremely long.It's all approximately exposure and intensity. Beyond that crimson line, hsps need to recharge.Getting the first-class from your surprisingly sensitive personalityA recluse decided he needed time far from the sector. He close himself inner a cave all alone and pondered. But soon the sound of dripping water in his sanctuary became unbearably loud. He was no happier inside the cave than out of doors it.The lesson here is that in case you're an hsp, you're going to want a few stage of flexibleness to discover, check, and regularly enhance your potential to control stimulation.Step one is to be type to your self. Deal with your mind and body as you would your little one self. Get right sleep, consume properly, exercising, and find a secure area you can constantly run to if you need to feel secure.That protection would possibly come within the form of deep, meaningful friendships with like-minded people who proportion your compassion for carrier, artwork, or spirituality.

Second, take into account that your frame will revolt at outdoor stress. Observe the direction a good way to lead you towards extra autonomy in such things as employment. Even at the same time as you're running for others, however, you could enhance the abilties to be able to ultimately buy your freedom.Excelling at your activity and communicating together with your superiors about what what works great for you may earn you greater flexibility.Constantly be touchy to bursts of creativity. Your instinct gives you foresight, making you good at evaluation and prediction in methods everyday human beings can't understand. However you should discover ways to prioritize to see initiatives via. Every other state of affairs you'll come upon is overall performance anxiety. Understand that this doesn't happen because you're shy or incompetent. In truth, about 30 percent of highly touchy human beings are extroverts, however still enjoy over-arousal.To combat performance anxiety, spend time on instruction, and pass into meetings or shows with notes to help you awareness.Don't forget, you need a social life as much as some other character. You simply need it in distinct doses. Assist your vast other and friends apprehend why you want a break but every now and then take some time to live out longer. This may lead them to happy, and has the delivered advantage of elevating your arousal threshold.Raising a sensitive child? Make sure they're securely connected. Give them the safety they want even as assisting them construct the confidence to exit and experiment.Meditation is an powerful way to calm hsps. Other than its recovery powers, meditation can transform beyond bad events into fine exchange.Say you purchased flustered at your first paintings presentation. Bear in mind the experience and your response. Became it disgrace, anger, or humilitaion?

Let your self sense that emotion. Don't withstand if your frame expresses it thru tears, rage or laughter.As an hsp, how can you are making it paintings next time for you. Remedy to take that step. Writing it down will make your remedy even more potent.Being type to your self, handling stimulation, training, correct conversation, and meditation will make you thrive as an hsp.Tremendously sensitive humans inherit nervous systems that are keener than those of the average character. This makes them experience, see, listen, take in, and procedure more facts from their surroundings.In case you enjoy a high level of stimulation, discover how your thoughts and body paintings. Deal with yourself with kindness, and progressively are seeking for autonomy in different aspects of your lifestyles. Domesticate significant relationships, move outside and play and recall: your superpower can be a gift to the sector.

Chapter 10. The history of a young Nigerian who cooks for hundred hours

History become made in lagos, nigeria, while hilda baci broke the guinness ebook of statistics, hitting a a hundred hours of cooking exclusive cuisine to the amazement of hundreds.For the target audience, who came to see a outstanding feat made and data smashed, it changed into certainly a rapturous environment at the amore gardens, lekki in lagos because the chef, on monday morning, smashed the 87 hours 45 mins document set with the aid of guinness international report holder, lata tandon.The 27-12 months-old has now broken the guinness world record for the longest cooking marathon with the aid of a man or woman as she clocked one hundred hours by using 8pm monday night time.Pronouncing her marathon cooking venture extension from ninety six to 100 hrs in an instagram publish on monday afternoon, baci's quality buddy @ama_reginald wrote: "'let's go. I requested my baby to make it a spherical discern, so we are doing 100hrs."As of 7:00 pm on monday, baci had cooked for ninety nine hours to surpass the previous report set with the aid of lata tondon, an indian chef, in 2019.Lata tondon cooked for 87 hours, forty five mins, and 00 seconds to break the previous title.Baci began her cooking marathon mission four days in the past at amore gardens.She will maintain cooking to extend the file till the hundredth hour.It's miles believed that once a man or woman has finished a document attempt, he/she must publish the proof to the frame.The first step for any successful guinness global information name holder is the fine in their application.Additionally, the period of time for the software procedure after which the evidence reviewed for the strive itself are taken into consideration.Guinness world file on its internet site stated: "the second one degree of the utility method occurs after your strive has taken location and requires you to put up your proof to us for assessment."once you have submitted your proof for a report try, there can be an proof overview length. The timeframe for this level will even depend on the sort of utility you've got opted for."it can take up to twelve weeks for us to check your documentation and let you know if your document try has been prevalent as the new record holder or rejected."

Hilda baci got colossal aid from celebrities, which include tiwa savage, kate henshaw, shawn faqua, to name some; they had been bodily present to hail the queen chef.Senator godswill akpabio and other senators-select this morning additionally paid a cohesion go to hilda baci as she set a new world record for the longest cooking marathon.Akpabio who occurs to be the previous governor of her state of origin, akwa ibom state, became visible having a flavor of hilda's meal in a video alongside saliu mustapha and other senators.Document-breaking nigerian chef, hilda bassey effiong, popularly called hilda baci, has narrated her experience in the contest in which that she shattered world information cooking for a hundred hours.She stated that it was not smooth making it into the guinness e-book of information, as she nearly gave up six hours into the competition.The graduate of sociology from madonna college who got here out from the restaurant after completing the a hundred-hour mark changed into complete of gratitude to god and those who gave her support, specially her mum and brother.For hilda's mum, mrs lynda ndukwe, her pleasure knew no bounds as she persevered to provide praises and glory to god. The proud mum referred to that she become grateful to god and all who stood by way of her.Ndukwe who got here from a humble background said there was a time she ought to best find the money for a one-room condominium in abuja however god has became things around, even extra now with the aid of the fame her daughter has gotten by using shattering the report books.She thanked famous cleric and revivalist, pastor jerry eze, who said her daughter's quest might end in praise.Ndukwe who is also a cook dinner and the leader executive officer of calabar pot has been a pillar of support to her daughter on the grounds that she began the cooking marathon.

Specific visuals of her were seen on-line, kneeling down in thanksgiving to god.Pmb, osinbajo, others rejoice as chef baci hits a hundred hours, makes guinness global document In the meantime, president muhammadu buhari has also shared the pleasure of celebrations with hilda bassey effiong, aka hilda baci, for making records by breaking the sector document of longest hours of cooking, locating her manner into the guinness book of records, and putting nigeria on the global highlight.Buhari, in a statement via presidential spokesman, femi adesina, lauded the younger culinary professional for turning her talent and ardour right into a profession, with a rippling effect on the economic system.He said hilda who runs a eating place in lagos, and trains different abilties on entrepreneurship, and now leads the arena in resilience, perseverance, and consistency in cooking.The president stated the antecedents of the restaurateur he said who dazzled on the jollof face-off opposition, 2021, preparing mouth-watering dishes that gained the selection prize, and settled an age-long contention with ghana on which african united states of america have to very own the trademark for cooking higher jollof-rice.Buhari expressed believe that hilda baci's drive and ambition have delivered more hobby and perception into the individuality of nigerian meals, as another cultural icon, with large tourism benefits, while he was hoping that more younger people will follow in her footsteps.The president thanked the sponsors of hilda baci cook dinner-a-thon, government officials, which includes governor babajide sanwo-olu of lagos state, celebrities from the effervescent music and movie enterprise, and lovers of the chef for all of the aid that has brought glory to the united states of america.Also, akwa ibom nation governor, udom emmanuel of akwa ibom state, sunday nighttime, reached out to miss hilda baci, commending her for representing the exceptional attributes of the dakkada (arise) philosophy of the kingdom.The governor, who joined different leaders, inclusive of the president-pick, asiwaju bola tinubu; vice president, yemi osinbajo; senator godswill akpabio, and lagos state governor, sanwolu, who in my view visited the lekki occasion centre to pat the worldwide chef on the lower back, the previous day dispatched a excessive -powered authorities delegation led via the commissioner for tourism, orman esin, to inspire her.Those legendary heroes belong to a princely elegance current in an early level of the history of a humans, and that they go beyond ordinary guys in skill, electricity, and braveness. They are commonly born to their role. A few, just like the greek achilles and the irish cú chulainn (cuchulain), are of semidivine foundation, unusual beauty, and super precocity. A few, just like the anglo-saxon beowulf and the russian ilya of murom, are darkish horses, slow to broaden.

Chapter 11.Experience a horror traditional, reanimated

Admit it you without delay have a photo in mind: a inexperienced, human like monster with bolts in its head. You furthermore mght in all likelihood understand that inside the authentic story, frankenstein isn't always without a doubt the call of the monster. It's the name of the scientist who creates the monster. However did you realize that the authentic book become written as early as 1816 did you aware of it turned into written through a woman and did you realize that mary shelley turned into just 18 years old whilst she came up with the story.That's not all that could marvel you about this horror traditional. On this e book, we'll take a deep dive into frankenstein to apprehend what makes it such a groundbreaking paintings of fiction.In case you want to study a exquisite short precis of the e book, you can bypass ahead to the final segment.

The loss of life of victor frankenstein

The story of frankenstein begins offevolved with four letters, written with the aid of an ambitious more youthful explorer named robert walton to his sister margaret. Walton recounts his preparations for his exploration venture to the north pole. Despite the fact that he reviews feeling lonely and isolated from his shipmates, he's pushed by means of his choice to accomplish a few issue first-rate. Speedy after setting sail, walton and his crew encounter a stranded, emaciated man caught inside the ice together together with his sledge. They take him on board and nurse him lower back to energy. In flip, the stranger stocks his tale.

He seems to be none apart from victor frankenstein.Victor starts offevolved offevolved the tale of his lack of lifestyles along together with his adolescence. He grows up because the only toddler of his nicely-to-do dad and mom in geneva. At the same time as he's five, his mother adopts an orphan lady, elizabeth. Aside from his quality buddy henry, elizabeth turns into victor's maximum cherished adolescence partner. Later, his mother and father have some different toddler, his more youthful brother william. From a young age, victor is obsessed on herbal philosophy. He mainly loves old university alchemists like cornelius agrippa, paracelsus, and albertus magnus. In the future, he watches a lightning bolt damage a tree near his residence and turns into focused on power.After his mom's untimely loss of life, 17-12 months-vintage victor leaves to have a study in ingolstadt, germany. His new professors update his scientific information and depart a deep impact with him. Victor is greater determined than ever to dedicate his existence to the pursuit of clinical greatness. Soon, he turns into so absorbed in his research that he forgets all about his circle of relatives in geneva. He's specially interested by the mysteries of life, loss of lifestyles and rot. However he goes further than every person before him: victor frankenstein discovers the secret of existence.

Analysis

Mary shelley started writing frankenstein in 1816, at the same time as she became simply 18 years antique, on a wet summer holiday inside the swiss alps. Trapped interior reading ghost tales, she and her journey partners started a horror tale contest. Among the ones companions were her destiny husband percy bysshe shelley, in addition to lord byron. But mary emerge as the first-rate one to later publish her story. The lifestyle of communal story-telling liable for the e book's introduction is meditated in its form. The story is especially informed thru explorer robert, who in turn hears it from frankenstein himself. But frankenstein's account too is interspersed with letters by means of manner of his circle of relatives. In a later a part of the e book, we even pay attention from the monster itself. So like every appropriate horror tale, the story of frankenstein is informed and retold typically. Mary shelley's travels to geneva and burg frankenstein in germany appear to have inspired the settings of the book. There's moreover a clean have an effect on of the gothic and romantic literary traditions of her time. However the combination of technological knowledge and horror she concocted changed into groundbreaking. A lot so that a few keep in mind frankenstein to be the first technological know-how-fiction novel of all time. "i'm able to pioneer a new way, find out unknown powers, and spread to the area the deepest mysteries of advent.

The introduction of frankenstein's monster

By way of now victor is spending all of his time in his condo, working on a mystery introduction to deliver to existence: a human-like creature with yellow skin, black hair and black lips. He grows so light and sickly over all this paintings that his family is seriously involved about him. However he gained't be deterred.In the end, on a rainy november night time, he animates his advent. However things don't flip out as expected. Victor has attempted to choose the creature's useless elements for beauty, however he's horrified on the ugly monster that involves life. He flees his apartment and spends the night out of doors. Within the city, he runs into his old pal henry, who has just arrived to examine on the university. Henry accompanies the traumatized victor again to his condo. However the monster is long past. Several months pass, in which henry nurses the shell-shocked victor returned to fitness. As soon as recovered, victor suggests henry across the college. However enticing with herbal technology now makes him especially nauseous. Victor's orphan-sister elizabeth sends a letter informing him that justine moritz, a woman who used to stay with their circle of relatives, has again to the house. A touch later, his father writes with some terrible information. His youngest brother william has been murdered. Victor leaves for geneva straight away. Within the woods outside the metropolis in which they located his brother's body, victor has an eerie encounter. He sees the monster lurking at the back of some trees, and becomes convinced that his advent is responsible for the murder. But the townspeople think the assassin is justine. Victor attempts to persuade them otherwise, however justine confesses to the crime out of worry. She's executed, and victor turns into ill with guilt.

Evaluation

On the coronary heart of frankenstein is a cautionary story approximately the risks of gambling god. Victor is so consumed via his clinical ambition that he neglects his family and friends. However he also fails to do not forget the effects and ethical implications of his grand experiment. Handiest after bringing the monster to life does victor recognize his grave mistake. But in preference to taking duty for his introduction, he runs faraway from it. Accordingly, the monster reasons the dying of of his beloved own family members. Victor realizes too late how lots chaos he's added into this world. However will he be able to accurate it.

The monster's curse

After william's and justine's loss of life, victor turns into so depressed that he even contemplates suicide. In hopes to cheer him up, his father takes the frankenstein family on a ride to their vintage home in switzerland. There, victor comes to a decision to climb the montanvert glacier to restore his naturalist spirit. But when he reaches the summit, the monster seems, jumping at him with "superhuman" speed. Victor curses and threatens his introduction, trying to persuade it to go away. However the monster eloquently appeals to victor's responsibility as its creator, and convinces him to comply with it into an ice cave.

Sitting through the fireplace, frankenstein's monster recounts the events of his life. It tells victor approximately the confusion and fright it felt upon being created, and the loneliness and depression it's skilled ever when you consider that. Since fleeing victor's apartment, it has wandered the desert, nearly pushed mad with the aid of starvation, thirst and cold. Each human it tries to technique runs away in terror.The monster eventually discovers a way to make fireplace, and is capable of preserve itself by stealing meals from human beings's houses. But upon looking at one of the poor families it's been stealing from, it starts offevolved to feel responsible. It tries to assist the circle of relatives by gathering firewood for them and leaving it on their doorstep. It also learns the names of its unwitting hosts – felix, agatha and their blind vintage father delacey – and starts offevolved growing a deep affection for them. When a overseas woman named safie joins the house, the monster is capable of choose up its resident's language along her. From eavesdropping on conversations, the monster learns approximately world occasions and the personal records of the cottagers. It also finds a bag of books containing john milton's paradise lost. No longer knowing that it's a work of fiction, the monster is deeply affected by the biblical story of the autumn of man. It's turning into an increasing number of disgusted by using its own ugliness and the unnatural way wherein it become created. In a closing wish to join the human network, the monster decides to show itself to the cottagers. It makes a plan to approach blind old delacey first, by myself. However because it's explaining its situation to him, felix, agatha and safie return to the cottage. Terrified by means of the monster's appearance, felix drives it away. After this sour rejection, the monster vows revenge on humankind however specially on its author victor. It travels for months to reach victor's domestic in geneva. Within the woods outside the town, the monster meets victor's younger brother, william. When he introduces himself as a frankenstein, the monster flies right into a rage and strangles him.

Evaluation

One of the maximum exciting and novel accomplishments of frankenstein is that components of the tale are told by using the monster itself. Mary shelley doesn't simply paint frankenstein's advent as a soulless ghoul reason on evil. At the opposite the monster is wise, eloquent, and really perceptive of human emotions. It's also certainly capable of affection, and desires not anything extra than to enroll in the human network. But the humans it encounters can't see beyond its devilish appearance. The monster is deeply pained via the worry and rejection hurled at it especially by using its personal writer. It's the ache of loneliness that in the long run drives it to emerge as violent. But even though it explains this to victor, and yet again appeals to his obligation as its writer, its message is lost on him as we'll see in the subsequent element. "all guys hate the wretched; how, then, need to i be hated, who am miserable past all living things.

The monster's bride

After telling its tale, the monster gives victor with a solution. It asks him to create a woman accomplice to ease its loneliness and isolation. This, the creature guarantees, might prevent it from being violent. It would disguise with its monster bride somewhere deep inside the jungle, by no means to be visible once more. Victor refuses inside the starting, however the monster ultimately convinces him. When they detail, but, victor places the concept of creating a monster bride on keep. He's however occupied collectively along with his grief over the dearth of william and justine. Plus, he's about to get married to elizabeth. However he speedy realizes that he can't accomplish that during actual experience of right and wrong with out pleasing his promise to the monster first. He asks his father to set up a -yr excursion of england, at some stage in which he plans to gather all the statistics needed to create the monster bride. His pal henry accompanies him on the travels. At the same time as they arrive in a small metropolis in scotland, victor comes to a decision to leave henry inside the care of an acquaintance. He travels to a desolate island in the orkneys, in which he sets up a small laboratory in a shack to finish the rest of his challenge in solitude. Simply due to the fact the primary time, victor is fed on with the useful resource of his work at the present day creature. However this time, there's no joy or excitement in it. He's ill to his belly about the horror he's developing. And he's concerned that the woman monster might not want to cover away in the jungle, or worse, that she'll want to have youngsters – spawning a "race of devils" inside the global.As he's taking into consideration this, he appears up at a window of his shack and sees the monster grinning at him. Taken aback via the sight of what he perceives to be pure evil, victor locks himself inside the shed and destroys his lady advent. The monster is furious. However in location of attacking victor right away, it sincerely offers him an eerie caution: it'll be there on his wedding ceremony night.

Analysis

One amazing challenge count number in frankenstein is the concept of obligation – specifically the responsibility of the writer to their creation. The monster regularly appeals to victor's obligation as its maker. It believes that as the person that has brought it to life, victor need to play some aspect in making that existence clearly worth living. For the motive that monster believes that its negative actions are the result of loneliness, it needs that victor create a associate for it. And even though he to begin with consents, victor is once more deterred with the aid of the hideousness of his advent. It's victor's superficial rejection of his introduction, and his refusal to deliver on his guarantees, that leads the monster to come to be genuinely evil.

unpleasant residue

Victor assembled his laboratory, crossed the ocean in his boat, and dropped the female creature's carcass into the water. Exhausted, he falls asleep and nearly drifts into the sea. Fortunately, the wind changed and he was able to reach dry land.

However, upon returning to the village, he never received a warm welcome. He learns that Henry has been killed and the townspeople believe him to be the killer. Some of them testified against him, claiming that he saw a boat similar to his on the night of the murder. When the town judge takes him to see Henry's body, Victor is shocked to see black marks on his neck from the monster's stranglehold. He faints and wakes up in prison, only to again fall ill with a mysterious illness. His father hurries from Geneva to be with him. He stays with Victor until trial, but is eventually acquitted. The Frankenstein family can return to Geneva. Victor is still determined to marry Elizabeth, but the monster's threat looms over his head. When the day of the wedding finally arrives, he becomes unbearably nervous.The couple spend their wedding night at his family's villa. Finally Victor lost his patience. He orders Elizabeth to sleep and begins searching her house for monsters. Suddenly you hear Elizabeth screaming.Too late, he realizes that the monster didn't try to kill him, but Elizabeth. Victor was shocked by her death and his father died a few days later in grief.Now Victor's entire family has been ruined by his own creation. He decides all that's left is to find and destroy the monster. His hunt takes him deep into the northern ice floes, where Walton and his team finally find him. Frankenstein ends as it began with a letter from explorer Robert Walton to his sister. Walton tells Victor that he is on his deathbed and encourages him to continue hunting monsters. However, Walton's team pleads with him to abandon the dangerous ice mission and return to England. Victor tries to persuade them to continue their ambitious quest, but Walton ends up listening to his men. Victor died shortly before the ship returned to England. A few days later, Walton hears strange noises coming from the room where Victor's body is kept. He investigates and is shocked to find a monster crying at Victor's bedside, thinking of its creator. However, he is too curious to attack. The monster tells Walton of his pain and regret for his wrongdoing. He tells her that now that her creator is dead, she is ready to die too. In the final scene, the monster bids farewell to Walton and disappears into the dark, cold ice.

analysis

Frankenstein is a story of boundless ambition, unethical science, and the dangers of the destructive power of loneliness. Victor's obsession with scientific fame first isolates him from his friends and family, eventually destroying them completely. Rejecting her outright, he leads his monstrous creation to evil. To make matters worse, Victor seems unable to learn from his mistakes. Even on his deathbed, he encouraged Walton and his team to continue their dangerous mission for the glory of science. Victor describes himself as misguided, superficial, and cowardly. He played God's part in the creation of life, but he doesn't want to play that part when it matters. In the final moments of his life, he became so inhuman that he considered himself a monster."I will die, and what I know now will no longer be felt. Soon this burning pain will disappear.my soul rests in peace. And if he thinks, of course he doesn't. separate.

Finally

Frankenstein tells the story of an ambitious scientist of the same name who is obsessed with the idea of creating life. But when young Victor Frankenstein finally manages to bring his work to life, he is struck by the horror he has created. Instead of taking responsibility, he leaves himself to the monster and runs away.This monster is not without mind and emotions, but is constantly rejected by human society. Eventually, his loneliness becomes unbearable and he vows revenge on his creator. He kills Victor's brother William, which leads to the execution of his girlfriend Justin. In a last-ditch attempt to stop its destruction, the monster asks Victor to make allies to ease his loneliness.But Victor again evades responsibility. As a result, he loses his best friend Henry, his childhood friend and future wife Elizabeth, and finally his father. A devastated Victor vows to hunt down and kill the monster. A chase takes him deep into the North, where he is picked up by young explorer Robert Walton, who ends up writing the story of Frankenstein's death.

Chapter 12.Discover the inspiring story of survival behind the innovation

Kyiv, March 14, 2022. As a crew of Fox News reporters were returning from the morning news, a second bomb blew up a vehicle near a combat zone. After a while, only two people survived.There was only one left before the burning wreckage of their car could be seen on the road.This Book follows the story of surviving journalist Benjamin Hall and a team of experienced professionals on an impossible mission to not only keep him alive, but also to get him out of Ukraine. Read on to learn what it takes to report on the front lines of global conflict.

voice in the dark

The first bomb detonated a clump of birch and pine trees 20 meters away. After a chaotic scene, veteran cameraman Pierre Zakrzewski shouted at the driver to change course, but the second bomb went off before anyone could react. In the silence and darkness after the second explosion, correspondent Benjamin Hall is running out of time. He felt no pain, no rush, nothing. Gradually, he noticed a familiar face in front of him. Then I heard my daughter's voice telling me to get out of the car. When she felt his presence, she realized she had to move if she wanted to live.Shocked and shocked, she did everything she could to get out of the back seat of the car in time. A moment later the third bomb exploded.Miraculously, Ben survives a bomb that destroys a small red car used by a Fox News crew that had recently arrived weeks earlier to cover the Russian invasion of Ukraine. His colleague Pierre also survived, but lay on the floor bleeding from a damaged femoral artery.Their situation was dire. The fighting was close, and the surroundings, far from the reporter's house in central Kiev, were deserted. As Ben regains consciousness and passes out again, he realizes that his injuries are serious. He also noticed that their car rolled along the main road and was unable to see it from the road to see if the car was passing. If he had any hope of salvation, he needed someone's attention. So he slowly began to climb up to be seen.After what seemed like hours, Ben finally heard a familiar sound. A car is approaching. In a last flash of strength, he waved wildly, screamed, and even threw bits of dirt at everything to get her attention. Soon he felt a hand grab the back of his coat and lift him up. In the blinding wave of pain that followed, his brain could only conceive of one thought. that they were saved.

Waking up

Ignorant of who had plucked his damaged frame off the roadside, ben remembers most effective fragmented photos of what accompanied. Rumbling along within the back of a van, and then some type of ambulance, he stored mumbling his call – that he was a journalist and an american, fearing he was in the arms of the russians. Then he saw a hypodermic needle being jabbed into his arm, and he exceeded out.He recalls a group of medical doctors soaring over him wearing headlamps, their swimming pools of light sweeping throughout his frame as they worked fast without energy. Subsequent, he become waking up in a clean, bright health facility mattress, convinced he was in russian palms. Terrified and questioning the nurses ought to be spies, ben felt trapped interior a cold struggle nightmare – until an american man walked over to his mattress and softly asked him his name, and whether or not or no longer he'd like to leave.What ben didn't recognize is that from the moment his crew had failed to test in numerous hours earlier, his colleagues in ukraine and abroad had sprung into motion. From an ocean away, the leader countrywide safety correspondent for fox information, jen griffin, had heard information that a group could have been hit at the outskirts of kyiv numerous hours in advance. Alerted through a colleague from agence france-presse, she first had to verify the tale, then training session a plan for what to do.Till getting gravely injured in a struggle area, ben didn't must keep in mind how he might be extracted if something went terribly incorrect. Entering into ukraine at the beginning of the warfare turned into exceptionally smooth. But because the millions of refugees at the pass in those early days can attest, getting overseas was gradual and exhausting. All of the buses have been packed for weeks with civilians fleeing the fighting, and educate strains have been being bombed as high-value objectives. Checkpoints have been thrown up everywhere, nearly in a single day. Neighborhood, basically inexperienced defense force had also made roadblocks, hoping to seize russian spies. America authorities had already evacuated its citizens, and issued the authentic word that every one civilians in ukraine after evacuation have been essentially on their very own. So even as surviving the preliminary bombing became fabulous, getting ben in a foreign country to be handled for his injuries turned into going to take a complicated series of extra miracles to drag off. Fortunate for him, this wasn't the primary time a person had needed to be extracted from a battle quarter, and there have been specialists who had been experts in getting them out.

on the road

She was safe, but Ben was in bad shape. Part of his right leg was immediately amputated. However, like his right arm, his left leg was badly damaged by the explosion. He knew he had been burned once, but he didn't know the severity of the burn. His eye was also cut in half by shrapnel, a skull fracture crushed his brain and he suffered several internal injuries in addition to shock.Even if it had been fine, getting Ben to the Polish border would have been difficult. Leaving the hospital in such a delicate state was dangerous for him.But at Fox News, Jen Griffin has been busy. After contacting the State Department to get emergency permission for survivors to leave Ukraine, she called her friend Sarah Verardo, founder of a unique organization called Save Our Allies (SOA). The group specializes in combat casualty rescue and was involved in rescuing 20,000 Afghan civilians from airports during the withdrawal of US troops in 2021. Sarah had a network of former military and humanitarian strategists in Ukraine trying to find and eliminate the team. He immediately thought of an agent named Seaspray who had returned to a venereal disease center in Poland after rescuing two Ukrainian girls. When the war broke out, they were left without their families in Ukraine and had to find them, eventually making their way to Poland.Sea Spray quickly found Ben and found him the sole survivor. The mission was modified slightly by notifying the families of the flight attendants who failed. Now they had to rescue Ben to safety despite his fragile condition and return cameraman Pierre Zakrzewski's body to his family. Seaspray also has a former Navy surgeon and honorary veteran, Dr. Rich Jedik, who was able to provide medical assistance along the way.Together they bought two old ambulances, filled them with volunteers, dressed in discreet medical suits and drove to Kiev. A battle-hardened leader, Syspray has completed hundreds of these missions and understands how to navigate the chaos of a war zone. I walked slowly through the back roads and fields, avoiding checkpoints as much as possible. They showed no signs of aggression or aggression towards anyone in the process and behaved as if they had every right to go where they were going.So Rich and Seaspray manage to get into the hospital where Ben is being treated and into his room on the third floor. It was Rich's voice asking Ben what his name was and if he wanted to go. The mission has officially begun.

An extended haul

Though ben's circumstance changed into essential, wealthy and seaspray had been capable of convince ukrainian doctors to discharge him. His circumstance was a ways worse than the already-beaten medical institution ought to deal with, and the various maximum vital interventions needed to be finished within forty eight hours of damage. The medical institution itself changed into also under regular danger from russian bombing; it couldn't assure that absolutely everyone would be safe within its partitions.

Rich and seaspray couldn't screen the other purpose they had to pass ben fast. They'd learned thru back channels that a diplomatic train sporting the top minister of poland became in kyiv for a assembly with ukrainian leaders. The educate sported heightened safety and wouldn't need to skip via bombed-out roads. It supplied the most secure, smoothest way overseas. The best trouble? They didn't have permission to tour at the train yet. But they also needed to get ben throughout the town to the main kyiv station, into the quite secured building, and onto the fairly guarded train.At the clinic, the crew turned into joined by using the fox information safety fixer who'd been helping them, nicknamed jock. Together, they bundled ben onto a gurney and into one of their ambulances, and waited for information from the polish embassy. Backstage, seaspray's operatives in poland were applying stress via diplomatic channels. In the meantime, motion throughout and out of kyiv became being in addition restricted. Greater checkpoints sprang up as a shoot-on-sight travel curfew became imposed. More and more, seaspray understood that the diplomatic train turned into the best way out, and made the decision to start traveling to the station while they awaited phrase. The educate would depart for poland whenever diplomatic talks ended, and that they had to be on it earlier than then.In poland and america, the diplomatic push became in complete pressure. A fellow soa operative became sending pics of ben's children to the polish diplomatic workplace. Other operatives had been clearing the manner in advance, alerting checkpoint after checkpoint approximately the ambulance sporting an injured american journalist. It somehow labored – soldiers let the ambulance skip. At the educate station, truly repeating the phrases american and scientific at the same time as smiling additionally worked; they had been allowed to enter the station and method the teach. As though on cue, they'd received reliable permission to journey almost concurrently. All that remained was getting ben onto the teach and right into a berth. Regardless of being in transit for hours with out food or ache medicinal drug, ben handiest asked for one issue in the train – his cell phone, in order that he should name his wife and daughters.

Surviving survival

By the time the educate began rumbling closer to poland, the ache medicinal drug ben were for the motive that morning in the health center become carrying off. He discovered on that train that his colleagues, cameraman pierre, and nearby interpreter, sasha, had died in the blast. Getting to poland have become additionally just the primary a part of what may be an extended adventure towards the medical facts ben needed to live on his blast accidents. Compound traumas like his had been uncommon outside of fight, and required professional care. Getting this care would possibly suggest visiting similarly than poland.

Back at fox records, the team had prepared a army pickup for ben. A helicopter could meet the teach and shipping ben first to a neighborhood polish military health facility. The personnel there would possibly then prepare him for the onward flight to a specialised scientific middle. For nearly forty eight hours, ben's high-quality idea had been to continue to exist. Now that he become secure and underneath navy medical remedy, he realized he was on a brand new journey.His injuries have been assessed as grave in ukraine, but it have become poland's procedure to catalog their proper volume, stabilize him, administer noticeably vital pain medicine, and get him on a quick flight from poland to the neighborhood clinical center at landstuhl, germany. Close to ramstein air base, and the headquarters of the usa air pressure in europe, this staff had massive understanding.Simply four days after the initial blast, ben become far from out of the woods. His giant burns made him vulnerable to infections that would kill him. His amputated leg became not an trouble, however the special leg had additionally been in component blown aside; the calf muscle changed into long past, and 1/2 of his foot have become missing. Saving this limb might be a mission, however it can make all the distinction in phrases of ben having the capability to walk again the usage of prosthetics. His broken eye needed to be eliminated, and he nonetheless had a beaten skull and brain harm.Healing, regardless of the exceptional clinical intervention, modified into going to be a much more laborious journey than crossing kyiv and leaving ukraine. The first-rate estimate have become at the least years. That's two years of additional surgical processes, collectively with painful pores and pores and skin grafts for his burns; years of bodily rehabilitation; and being fitted and refitted for prosthetic limbs. It intended studying to walk over again – and mastering the manner to navigate the arena along with his new physical barriers, so he may need to go back to being the active father and husband his family had normally acknowledged him to be.

The road home

One of the excellent alternatives for such lengthy-time period care turned into on the brooke military medical middle, in texas. However getting there has been going to take extra grit – and a lengthy flight in a army c-17 cargo aircraft without pain remedy, so he'd stay alert. Knowing he had no preference, ben set his solve and got through the ache one extra time.

Even as the health workers had expected two years of treatment and rehabilitation, benjamin corridor turned into decided to make this technique faster. Tons faster. All of the efforts by way of his group, colleagues, and the diplomats, navy specialists, and clinical team that had ensured his survival stimulated him to take on his recovery with zeal and cause. He cheerfully faced surprising setbacks, painful interventions, and incessant physical demanding situations in honor of those who had come to his aid. Understanding his colleagues hadn't survived meant ben's healing was in their names as properly. On this spirit, ben honestly left brooke military medical middle just five months after arriving in texas. He waved goodbye to the body of workers he'd come to cherish and boarded a plane again home – marveling on the knowledge that had now not only repaired his body, however given him a future with his own family.Even when journalist Benjamin Corridor's news team was attacked early in the conflict in Ukraine, the survival of the improvised bomb was astonishing. The concerted effort required to preserve it, treat it scientifically, and bring it safely abroad was expert personnel, diplomatic and military cooperation, and many fortunate corporations. Realizing the incredible happiness, Ben accepted everything to bring his family home.

Heroes are competent and confident

It takes both skill and self-self belief to rush into wherein others fear to tread. Researchers advocate that folks that perform heroic acts tend to experience assured in themselves and their skills.While faced with a disaster, they've an intrinsic notion that they're capable of coping with the mission and accomplishing achievement irrespective of what the percentages are. A part of this self belief might stem from above-common coping skills and abilities to control pressure.Heroes aren't afraid to face fear.A person who rushes right into a burning building to shop another man or woman isn't just pretty brave; she or he additionally possesses an capacity to overcome fear. Researchers propose that heroic individuals are advantageous thinkers via nature, which contributes to their capacity to appearance past the immediate threat of a state of affairs and spot a extra optimistic final results.In many cases, those individuals may additionally have a higher tolerance for danger. Lots of caring and type people might shy away within the face of chance. Individuals who do jump into motion are typically more likely to take more dangers in more than one elements of their lives.Heroes hold working on their dreams, even after multiple setbacks. Endurance is some other quality typically shared by means of heroes.When confronted with a potentially life-threatening contamination, people with heroic dispositions would possibly awareness on the best that would come from the state of affairs which includes a renewed appreciation for existence or an accelerated closeness with cherished ones.The selection to behave heroically is a preference that a lot of us can be referred to as upon to make at some point in time. By means of conceiving of heroism as a time-honored attribute of human nature, now not as a unprecedented characteristic of the few 'heroic opt for,' heroism turns into some thing that seems within the range of opportunities for anyone, perhaps inspiring greater of us to reply that call," write heroism researchers, zeno franco, and philip zimbardo.Constructing empathy, becoming able and professional, and being continual in the face of limitations are all competencies you may paintings on through the years. Via doing so, you can enhance your capability to help others and come through in times of need.In wonder films together with captain the us: the primary avenger, the "hero" of the storyline is an attractive guy, pumped up like a balloon with superhuman quantities of steroids.Word: i distinctly revel in this movie, however the quantity of realism in its plot resembles my flames cash account at the end of the semester hardly some thing is gift.This storyline results in an expectation of receiving supernatural ability or success so one can be categorised as a "hero," when the characteristics of a hero are certainly discovered inside captain america via his willpower to army provider, strong will and courageous coronary heart.However for many people, heroes today are merely described by way of reputation, appearance, cash or ridiculous acts.The espys recent arthur ashe award for courage winner, caitlyn jenner, has maximum of the sector either enticed or enraged through her "heroic" deeds.

The arthur ashe award for braveness became given to jenner due to her display of "courage and self-reputation" according maura mandt, espys co-executive producer.The best trouble is the assessment among arthur ashe and caitlyn jenner.Arthur ashe, a champion tennis player and humanitarian was quoted on reaction capability's website, an company targeted on selling brave leadership, about his tackle heroism."authentic heroism is remarkably sober, very undramatic," the website quoted ashe. "it isn't the urge to surpass all others at some thing cost, but the urge to serve others at anything fee."Jenner's gender alternate regarded within the public eye for weeks.Did jenner's alternate serve other transgenders? Perhaps, however others may also now see the media as a platform to grab interest thru twitter favorites and fb shares.On this media-driven age, the heroes of these days are being driven behind people who do not match the description of a ashe's "hero."In mild of this current occasion, the word hero ought to be described.Via a compilation of definitions among merriam-webster and dictionary.Com, a hero is someone who is renowned for first-rate or courageous acts, fine characteristics, and having braveness or capability.The 3 american squaddies, the frenchman and the briton who stopped a gunman onboard a train aug. 21, in step with the richmond times—dispatch, have to be taken into consideration true heroes because of their selflessness in placing their lives on the line to protect others. They confirmed braveness and bravery in the face of a massive gun and a small danger of survival. They persisted besides, and that they requested not anything for the deed. They sincerely desired to guard others at some thing price.

Sounds greater like the ashe quote, proper?

Even supposing those squaddies cannot win an espy because they do now not without delay correlate to sports activities, they are still the authentic heroes. And to locate the true hero, we must now not appearance on the tv display or at the film theatres, however we have to look for those with selfless hearts, bravery, and the potential to guard and protect while no one is asking.Often, genuine heroes cover at the back of the normalcy of regular life, and to locate them, all we need to do is look.